Step by Step to Involving Parents in Health Education

David A. Birch, PhD, CHES

ETR ASSOCIATES
Santa Cruz, California
1996

ETR Associates (Education, Training and Research) is a nonprofit organization committed to fostering the health, well-being and cultural diversity of individuals, families, schools and communities. The publishing program of ETR Associates provides books and materials that empower young people and adults with the skills to make positive health choices. We invite health professionals to learn more about our high-quality publishing, training and research programs by contacting us at P.O. Box 1830, Santa Cruz, CA 95061-1830, 1-800-321-4407.

About the Author

David A. Birch, PhD, CHES, is an associate professor in the Department of Applied Health Science at Indiana University in Bloomington. He was formerly director of health education outreach programs in the Department of Health Education at Pennsylvania State University in University Park, Pennsylvania. He has extensive experience in developing and conducting teacher training programs in health education and has published numerous articles in professional journals. He serves as a member of the board of directors of both the Association for the Advancement of Health Education and the American School Health Association. He is currently a member of the editorial board of the *Journal of Wellness Perspectives* and is Continuing Education Editor of *Health Values*. He has also served as secretary of the Board of Commissioners of the National Commission for Health Education Credentialing. He has worked at the state level for the Maine Department of Educational and Cultural Services and has more than ten years of public school teaching experience.

Published by ETR Associates, P.O. Box 1830, Santa Cruz, California 95061-1830

Printed in the United States of America

10 9 8 7 6 5 4 3 2 1

Title No. H550

Birch, David A.
        Step by step to involving parents in health education /
    David A. Birch
                p.   cm.
        Includes bibliographical references (p. 113).
        ISBN 1-56071-474-3
        1. Health education—Parent participation—United
States.   2. Health education—
Parent participation—United States—Evaluation.
3. Teachers—In-service training—United States.
I. Title.
LB1587.P37B57   1996
372.3'7'0973—dc20   95-24324

Contents

Appendixes

     National Education Goals

     Assessment and Planning Process

     The 8 Components of a Comprehensive School Health Program

     Quotes to Spark Discussion

     Addressing Concerns About Family Involvement

Figures and Examples

Figures

Examples

Acknowledgments

I would like to thank my editor, Kathleen Middleton, for both her dedication to the improvement of comprehensive school health education, and her belief in the importance of parent involvement. Kathleen's guidance, patience and support were especially helpful during the development of this publication.

In addition, I would like to acknowledge the efforts of the many dedicated teachers, parents and family members who not only recognize, but fulfill the shared responsibility of helping children and teenagers reach their full potential.

Most important, I would like to thank my family for their ongoing love and support. To my mother, Virginia Birch, I express my appreciation for her example of living life to its fullest; and to Ruthann, Megan and Sarah, my appreciation for their understanding and patience during another health education project.

Preface

Although much time and effort are spent assessing instructional strategies in education, few are considered universally effective. One strategy that comes close to universal acceptance, however, is actively involving parents and other family members as partners in their children's education.

Researchers have found that "parent involvement is directly related to significant increases in student achievement" (Chavkin, 1989). The current emphasis on parent involvement is exemplified by the inclusion of "increased parent participation" as one of the eight goals in the Goals 2000: Educate America Act, which provides direction for educational reform for the rest of the decade.

This book offers step-by-step procedures and background information to help schools and health educators involve parents and other family and community members as partners in comprehensive health education. It emphasizes active, meaningful involvement directly related to instruction—involvement that goes beyond the traditional roles of classroom aides, parent organizations and volunteers for school projects. The following examples of family involvement illustrate the dynamic potential of successful programs:

- Several parents representing different segments of the community serve as members of the health education program development committee.

- The uncle and legal guardian of a high school student is a member of the school district health education materials review committee.

- Parents and other family members attend a weekly school-based class on cardiovascular health, which includes topics such as healthy meals and family exercise activities.

- Using flashcards, a grandparent reviews home safety rules with a second grader.
- A student and her parent read an article on a health issue covered in the high school health class and discuss personal and family values related to the issue.

This book provides direction for including parents and other family members in activities to enrich classroom instruction, with a focus on health-related issues. It includes a rationale for family involvement; descriptions of a variety of ways to involve families, including decision making, adult learning experiences and at-home activities; discussion of important issues around family involvement; and guidance for assessing and improving family involvement efforts.

The terms "family involvement" and "parent involvement" are used interchangeably throughout the book. Contemporary students live in a variety of family structures and situations and may not have parents who can participate in a partnership with the school. For these students, grandparents, aunts, uncles, siblings and other adults may be key individuals for involvement.

Collaboration between teachers, administrators and parents is critical at both the school and district levels. The potential of comprehensive school health education will not be reached without this essential partnership.

1

Families, Health and Schools

The interaction between parents and children may well be the most important key to lasting, long-term improvements in the overall health status of this country.
—James O. Mason

Family involvement is a win-win situation for all. Schools benefit, communities benefit, families benefit, but, most important, children benefit. Regardless of economic and social status, families and communities have high aspirations for their children. It is critical that schools and communities work together toward common goals. This means that parents and educators must be full partners.

The healthy growth and development of children is dynamic and interactive. The responsibilities of parents, teachers and community members often overlap. Generalizations can be made for responsibilities, but the bottom line is that children's educational success is related to their health status, which is related to their home situations.

The fact that education is a dynamic system involving schools, homes and communities is evident in the *Goals 2000: Educate America Act,* passed in 1994. (See Figure 1.) Goal 8 states *Schools will promote partnerships with parents to increase their participation in their children's education.*

The National Education Goals specifically require interaction outside the walls of the school. Issues of safety, adult literacy, children's health status and family involvement are considered as important as competency in specific content areas. This law encourages state departments of education and local school districts to increase parent and family involvement. It may also make federal funding available to help achieve the goals.

Figure 1

National Education Goals

1. Children will enter school ready to learn.

2. The high school graduation rate will be 90 percent.

3. Students will leave fourth, eighth and twelfth grades having showed competency in English, mathematics, science, foreign languages, civics and government, economics, arts, history and geography.

4. Teachers will have the professional development they need to help students reach the other goals.

5. American students will be first in the world in math and science achievement.

6. Every adult will be literate and have the skills to compete in the global economy and participate in American democracy.

7. Schools will be free of drugs, violence, unauthorized guns and alcohol.

8. Schools will promote partnerships with parents to increase their participation in their children's education.

Source: Hoff, D. 1994. Goals 2000 will shape state and local school reform. *Report on Education Research* 26 (12): 1–8.

Keys to Effective Programs

Families should be involved in all subject areas of the curriculum, at all grade levels as part of a districtwide effort. Schools must reach out and involve parents as legitimate partners in educational efforts. The traditional open house, PTA meetings, and parent bake sales, while important, are not sufficient to maximize family involvement.

Developing, promoting and sustaining a staff and family partnership requires commitment on the part of a school system.

This commitment should include the following steps:

1. Mission

Have a clear mission statement. Make it clear in the school philosophy or mission statement that parents and other family members are important partners in students' education.

2. Validation

Validate the partnership. School staff acknowledge and validate the worth and positive influence of people from all family structures and situations. This starts with a sincere desire to work as partners.

3. Communication

Communicate frequently. Encourage and model clear and frequent messages to family members about their possible roles and responsibilities as partners.

4. Planning

Involve families in planning. The families themselves are one of the best sources of ways parents and other family members can be involved. They should be included in the planning of any family involvement programs.

5. Programs

Provide specific programs for involvement. Design programs and resources to educate parents and other family members. Involve them in school decision making and in structured at-home activities that engage them as partners in their children's learning.

6. Inservice

Provide inservice training. Inservice training for teachers and other staff members helps them develop awareness of the importance of family involvement and the skills and resources needed to facilitate such involvement.

7. Time

Allocate time. Development, implementation and evaluation of family involvement activities require time. Teachers and other staff members should be allowed adequate time and resources.

8. Evaluation

Evaluate and revise. Evaluate all aspects of the school and district family involvement programs. Make adjustments and refinements based on the findings.

Comprehensive School Health Programs

The goal of creating healthy, educated children and youth requires the integration of educational systems with health and social systems. Leaders in school health education have identified ten topic areas that should be included in school health instruction.

The ten topic areas:

- mental and emotional health
- family life
- nutrition
- substance use prevention
- personal health and fitness
- disease prevention and control
- injury prevention and safety
- consumer health
- community health
- environmental health

School health education addresses from a prevention standpoint many severe problems that plague our nation and our nation's children. These include violence, drug use, teenage pregnancy and sexually transmitted disease (STD).

Health instruction should be one component of a broader school health promotion model known as the comprehensive school health program. (See Figure 2.) Family and community involvement is considered a foundational component in a comprehensive school health program (Allensworth and Kolbe, 1987). The effectiveness of school health education can be greatly increased when schools, parents and other family and community members work together to address critical health education issues.

Figure 2
The 8 Components of a Comprehensive School Health Program

School Health Instruction

In-class aspect of the program based on a planned and sequential curriculum. Interacts with the other components to enable young people to achieve optimal health.

Healthy School Environment

Physical and psychological surroundings of students, faculty and staff. The physical environment is free of hazards; the psychological environment fosters students' personal achievements and social growth.

School Health Services

Activities designed to appraise, protect and promote the health of students and school personnel, including preventing communicable disease and providing emergency care for injury or sudden illness.

Physical Education and Fitness

Opportunities for students to participate in daily physical activity, as well as exposure to information about how and why to partake in activities and encouragement to develop skills that contribute to lifetime fitness.

(continued...)

Figure 2 *(continued)*

The 8 Components of a
Comprehensive School Health Program

School Nutrition and Food Services

Opportunity to establish health norms and model healthy nutritional behaviors. Schools that provide healthy food choices send a clear message to students about the importance of good nutrition.

School-Based Counseling and Personal Support

Opportunity to respond to special needs and provide personal support for students, teachers and staff, as well as promotion of schoolwide mental, emotional and social well-being.

Schoolsite Health Promotion

Combination of educational, organizational and environmental activities designed to encourage students and staff to adopt healthier lifestyles and become better consumers of health care services.

School, Family and Community Health Promotion Partnerships

Collaborative efforts that share a common vision of healthy young people and focus on health promotion and disease prevention to solve communitywide threats to the future health of youth.

Why Family Involvement?

The positive outcomes of family involvement range from positively influencing children's behavior to meeting the needs and interests of parents.

An important first step in moving toward meaningful involvement is for both parents and school staff members to understand the rationale for family involvement. The following ideas can help form this rationale.

Influence

Family members can influence students' behaviors. Many factors affect the health-related decisions that people make. Health education occurs in the context of family, community, religion, media and other messages students receive about health. The quality of school health education can affect the health-related decisions that students make now and in the future. However, many other life experiences also influence health-related behaviors.

Students are heavily influenced by health choices family members make, in particular, the health behaviors modeled by their parents. Parents, other family members, school staff and community members all model health-related behaviors. Examples include:

- food selection and preparation
- alcohol and other drug use
- stress management
- communication
- physical activity

These behaviors, whether healthful or less healthy, help to establish a climate that influences children's health decisions.

Desire

Families want to be involved. The majority of parents want to be involved in their children's education. In studies of families from diverse ethnic and cultural backgrounds, researchers have found that more than 95% of parents express strong support for the idea of family involvement (Chavkin and Williams, 1985). Parents want to know more about helping their children learn and succeed. However, many parents feel that they do not get enough direction from schools and teachers in how to do so.

Health education opportunities can provide families with meaningful ways to be involved. Parents are concerned about the health and welfare of their children. Involvement activities designed to meet the needs and interests of family members may be the best and most successful way to involve them.

Personal Growth

Family members can increase their own personal health knowledge and skills. Many adults benefit from participating with their children in formal health education activities. Health education instruction where students and families work together at home on specific activities can help family members learn new information, examine health-related attitudes and develop skills.

Several studies have indicated positive changes in the health behavior of parents after participation in such activities. In an evaluation of a cardiovascular health education program, parents reported that their own food intake and exercise habits were healthier after the program than before (Hearn et al., 1992). A four-week, take-home drug prevention program led to increased parent/child communication about drug prevention and increased interest on the part of fathers in helping their children avoid drug use (Werch et al., 1991).

In a review of literature dealing with health-related behaviors in families it was concluded that children can influence the attitudes and behaviors of their parents (Perry, Crockett and Pirie, 1987). As one parent of an elementary school student said, "I become angry when my second grader informs me at the dinner table that I'm not serving him a balanced meal. I must admit that I am learning many nutritional facts from him" (Epps, 1987).

Reinforcement

Family members can provide reinforcement. Families can reinforce the information that students learn, the attitudes they form and the skills they develop in school health education programs. Possible reinforcement activities include:

- family members working together on a home health education assignment
- family members emphasizing healthful consumer behavior while shopping in a supermarket or pharmacy
- family members working together on a skill, such as preparing a low-fat meal or practicing a stress management technique or assertive communication

Family Perspective

Family members can present a family perspective on sensitive topics. Many of the topics in health education, such as family life and sexuality, HIV, substance use and abuse, and mental health, address issues related to family values. Sound health education enables and encourages parents, students and other family members to clarify family perspectives on these topics.

Structured discussions related to health topics between students and their families are critical. Family members also should be formally involved in curriculum decisions for health education. Districts should set up specific guidelines for this involvement process that promote a balanced and wide representation from the community.

Support

Families can lend support to a program. Involvement in family activities helps educate parents and other family members about comprehensive school health education. Family members who are educated and involved in school health education are more likely to be program supporters and advocates.

Positive Educational Effects

Family involvement has a positive effect on students. Educators generally agree on the positive effects of parental involvement. Much evidence links significant increases in school achievement to parental involvement. Studies of cooperative efforts between parents and educators have concluded that the home curriculum provides a better prediction of academic learning than family socioeconomic status (Walberg, 1984). Reported benefits include:

- academic achievement

- increased student attendance

- fewer student dropouts

- improvement in student self-achievement

- more parent and community support of the school

Benefits have also been found specific to health education. In a study of a fourth through sixth grade drug education program that included weekly family involvement assignments found that children in the program reported a more accurate perception of peer use of alcohol, tobacco and marijuana than students in a control group (Werch et al., 1991). This is important because students usually have a mistaken perception about the prevalence of drug use among peers. Actual use is much lower than students perceive.

Numerous studies confirm that family involvement promotes adoption of positive behaviors related to prevention of adolescent pregnancy, prevention of substance abuse and choosing appropriate nutrients (Allensworth, 1994). Other research on health education programs that include parent involvement indicates positive changes in smoking behavior among parents (Bernier, 1991), in parental eating and exercise habits (Hearn et al., 1992), and in child/parent discussion about health topics (Perry, Crockett and Pirie, 1987).

Barriers to Family Involvement

Family involvement isn't always easy. Parents, teachers, administrators and other school staff members may have limited experience with family involvement in school programs, especially in areas such as instruction and decision making. Family members may feel inadequate, uncomfortable or lack adequate direction from the school.

Some teachers and administrators may view parent involvement as a liability rather than an asset. They may not have been trained in the skills that help promote meaningful family involvement. School staff members may believe that many parents are not willing to be involved in their children's education.

Family involvement programs need careful planning and support—at both the individual school sites and district office. Teachers need to create new kinds of connections with parents and other community resources. They also need the support of school and district administrators for their efforts. Designing family involvement programs requires new and creative methods for:

- attracting family members to the school
- reaching family members at home
- engaging teachers in the use of family involvement activities to improve curriculum and instruction

However, when both family members and school staff understand the rationale and benefits of family involvement, the rewards of implementing an involvement program can be great. One principal of an inner-city school described both the frustrations and the rewards of a family involvement program in this way:

> Yes, we've still got problems getting parents involved. At times, it seems like we're climbing a hillside of shale. We take a few steps up and then slide back down. But we keep putting one foot ahead of the other, doing whatever works. We try to learn from our mistakes and to look at failure as a learning process. We'll keep trying until something finally works, and then we'll try to improve it.
>
> The bottom line is that, where we had practically nothing before, we now have something. Where we had a negative attitude and a feeling of hopelessness before, now we can actually see a bit of sun shining through the clouds (Bartell, 1992).

2

Working with Diverse Family Cultures

The whole village educates the child.

—African Proverb

The ethnic and racial profile of the United States population has changed and will continue to change as the country moves into the twenty-first century. Demographic changes expected by the year 2000 include increases in the populations of African Americans, Asians and Pacific Islanders, Hispanics, and Native Americans, including Alaskan Natives.

By the year 2000, one-third of the students in American schools will be members of the Asian-American, African-American, Hispanic or Native-American cultures. This diversity increases the importance of family involvement in health education. According to Hernandez and Day (1994), "Family involvement is particularly critical in multicultural settings where the variety of values, beliefs, attitudes, learning styles, and languages makes health education a challenge." Bensley (1994) states:

> The teacher's attitude toward teaching in a multiethnic setting is the first consideration in meeting the personal and professional challenge that can lead to satisfaction and confidence in his or her teaching abilities.

> Preparing oneself to teach in a multiethnic classroom demands an open mind and a positive attitude towards the beliefs and values of all groups.

Aspects of Family Culture

Race and ethnicity are not the only variables related to family culture. Family structure has also changed. Nearly half of the children in the United States live apart from one or both parents or with people other than their parents.

Other variables related to family culture:

- educational level
- religious background
- attitude toward education
- socioeconomic level
- aspirations
- multilingual proficiency
- access to transportation
- individual health behaviors

Effective family involvement efforts are designed to reach parents and family members living in a variety of family situations. An awareness and appreciation of differences in family structures, combined with individual and cultural respect and a vision of the potential of all families as partners in education, will promote successful family involvement efforts.

Working with Family Diversity

The following suggestions may help educators work more effectively with all parents and family members.

Culture

Learn about the cultures of children in the school system. Teachers and other school staff can become familiar with characteristics of the cultures represented by students and their families. Many cultures have unique perceptions of the family structure and the role of the extended family.

In some cultures, aunts and uncles or other relatives are considered "immediate family," serving in the same roles as parents in school activities. For example, in the Native American community, "elders" play key roles in family involvement activities because of the culture's respect for their wisdom.

The relationship of children to other family members and adults and the behavior of adult family members can affect school performance, interactions with school staff and family involvement efforts. An example of this type of cultural difference is the principle of "pride and shame" practiced by some Asian Americans. Related to school, this principle refers to the intense shame, guilt and anxiety suffered by a family if a child is referred to a school administrator or counselor (Morrow, 1991).

Families' previous experiences with schools and school staff will influence their attitudes about current family involvement efforts. Families from particular cultures may feel isolated from the school culture (Delgado-Gaitan, 1991). This isolation increases when schools promote family involvement activities that require knowledge about school and specific behaviors based on the majority culture.

Myths

Address the myth that certain families do not want to be involved. One potential barrier to family involvement efforts may be a perception on the part of school staff that some parents do not care about or do not want to be involved in their children's education.

However, research indicates that regardless of ethnicity, socioeconomic status, education, marital status or vocation, most parents do want to be involved. One significant barrier to involvement may be parental distrust of or discomfort in dealing with the school, which may be related to past experience or a perceived lack of skills.

Parents and other family members need to see that their involvement is valued. They need clear messages about the method and nature of their involvement. When parents who had been uninvolved become involved in their children's education, they develop a sense of self-efficacy that is passed on to their children (Figueroa, 1993).

Sensitivity

Avoid insensitive language. Beware of certain terms or phrases that reinforce stereotypes. For example, a statement such as, "Mary Baldwin, a bright, articulate, African-American mother from the West Side, is the chair of the family involvement task force," could be interpreted as suggesting that Baldwin is an exception when compared to other African-American women from the West Side. Another example is identifying a person by race or ethnic background when it is not appropriate, such as "a Hispanic principal." Similarly, descriptions of non-nuclear family structures as "broken homes" or of families living with socioeconomic limitations as "lower class" are stereotypical and demeaning.

Materials

Use culturally sensitive curriculum materials that depict individuals from all backgrounds. Curriculum materials that include references to and depict individuals from diverse cultural groups in a positive manner enhance the school's educational efforts. Providing these types of materials begins with the curriculum development process. When the people involved in curriculum development reflect the true composition of the school district community, the materials they select are likely to reflect this diversity as well.

A guide entitled *Criteria for Comprehensive Health Education Curricula*, published by the Southwest Regional Education Laboratory, provides an excellent resource for curriculum development. It contains scales to examine curriculum characteristics, including cultural equity.

A culturally sensitive health education curriculum has specific characteristics (Pahnos and Butt, 1994).

Characteristics of a sensitive curriculum:

- promotes values, attitudes and behaviors that support cultural pluralism
- reflects the cultural learning styles of all students
- fosters positive multicultural interactions between teachers and students
- develops skills necessary for both interpersonal and intercultural interaction
- uses assessment procedures that reflect students' cultural preferences

Communication

Minimize language barriers to effective communication. Language can often be a barrier to effective communication between school staff and family members. Communicating with family members who have limited English proficiency is a challenge that must be addressed by both staff and families. The following recommendations have been adapted for all languages from suggestions by Cooper and Gonzalez (1993) for communicating with Spanish-speaking parents.

Recommendations for communication:

- Be sure that at least one person on the school staff is fluent in languages spoken by students' families.

- Be sure that essential written materials are printed correctly in both English and other appropriate languages.

- Acquire translation devices, especially for large group presentations such as parent/teacher nights.

- Ask staff members to attempt to learn the languages spoken by students' families.

- Remain attentive, despite linguistic differences.

- Form parent advisory committees to examine ways of improving communication.

- Take the initiative in resolving problems.

- Respect all languages and cultures.

Another challenge related to communication has to do with verbal style. Some cultures may use a communication style that works well in their community or environment but is different from the communication style of the majority culture. This difference in style may lead to perceptions that people from this culture are less intelligent or less educated than others. Understanding the cultural environment reduces the chances that differing communication styles will be a barrier to effective communication.

Personal Choices

Be sensitive to health choices of family members. The behaviors of individuals within a family are one aspect of the family culture. As students learn about positive health practices and the consequences of unhealthy practices, they may become concerned about the health choices and behaviors of others, especially family members.

Some family members may engage in unhealthy behaviors, such as smoking, poor dietary habits, or alcohol or other drug use. These behaviors may present a conflict to students. When children express their concerns to these family members, some may respond negatively. Consequences can range from discomfort to abusive or even violent behavior.

Teachers and family members who are prepared can help children deal with these issues. A first step is keeping family members aware of the topics being covered in health education class so children's concerns can be anticipated. With this awareness, both teachers and family members can then explain to children that behaviors occur in the context of life situations and that some behaviors may be difficult to stop.

Tobacco use prevention education provides an example. A child who is involved in a unit on the dangers of smoking may feel anger toward a loving, responsible family member who smokes. Teachers who are aware that some children have family members who smoke can emphasize to students that smoking is a difficult habit to give up. They can emphasize ways to communicate concern and point out that family members who have an unhealthy habit may also have some very healthy habits.

Logistics

Consider logistical issues. Barriers to family involvement often result from logistical considerations. These considerations may involve lack of transportation, difficulty in leaving work or lack of childcare. Educators who are sensitive to these difficulties will find creative ways to work around these barriers to provide opportunities for family involvement activities.

Educators must be cognizant of the differences in the family cultures of their students. An awareness, and appreciation, of these differences, along with a vision of the potential of all families as partners, are necessary for successful family involvement efforts.

3

Family Involvement Strategies

Health education occurs in the context of family, community, religious and media messages concerning health.
—Maurice Elias

The best way to involve family and community members in educational efforts is as legitimate partners. Schools and educators have a responsibility to reach out to all parents to involve them both at home and at school in meaningful activities that contribute to the mission of the school.

Family and community members can be involved in many different activities at varying levels—from the individual classroom to district committees. Key avenues to family involvement include:

- decision-making responsibilities
- health education programs for family members
- at-home learning activities

Involving Families in Decision Making

Parent involvement in school decision making is a critical component of family involvement. Both educators and parents agree on its importance. Organizations such as the national Parent Teacher Association (PTA) have long worked toward the goal of involving families in school decision making.

Important areas for family involvement in decision making include **curriculum development** and participation on **health advisory committees and councils.**

Curriculum Development

A committee for curriculum development provides an excellent opportunity for family members to be involved in decision making related to school health education. On such a committee, family members work with administrators, teachers, other school staff, students and community members to develop the curriculum for the comprehensive school health program. They have the opportunity to provide input into curriculum decisions and interact with other committee members.

Family involvement in curriculum development benefits the school district by providing a family perspective on health education needs and parental input into decisions on health education content. This input is especially valuable in sensitive topic areas such as sexuality education.

In addition, family and community members who are involved in curriculum development have an investment in the curriculum and are more likely to support the health education program. This support is helpful to districts facing decreases in funding for health education and/or community opposition to the health education curriculum.

Inviting Involvement

Involvement in curriculum development begins with open invitations to all family and community members to participate on the committee itself. Announcements can be sent to all families in the form of a letter that describes the committee's focus and indicates how often committee meetings will occur. The announcement should also include a name and phone number people can contact for more information or to express their interest. (See Example 1.)

Example 1

Curriculum Development Committee

Dear Family:

The Hilltop School District is forming a committee to help plan the district's health education program. Parents and other family and community members are invited to serve on the committee along with school staff and students.

The Committee will meet once a month. Some work may be required outside of committee meetings.

If you are interested in becoming a committee member or would like further information contact _____ at 555-1234.

Thank you for your interest.

Announcements can be distributed in many different ways:

- sent home with students (not always the most reliable method)
- published in school newsletters
- mailed home with student report cards
- published in community newspapers
- posted in prominent community locations
- communicated as public service announcements on radio and television

Composition of the Committee

In effective programs, the composition of the committee reflects the composition of the community. No one group or one area of the school district has disproportionate representation.

An effective curriculum development committee is large enough to include key people but not so large that it hinders the decision-making process. When many family and community members are interested in participating on the committee, selection of committee members may present a dilemma. A balance must be struck between open participation and committee efficiency.

Larger, general community meetings can be held to allow for greater participation and generate broader input to the curriculum development committee. Such meetings provide opportunities for more family and community members to be involved in the process. Locations of these meetings should be accessible to all members of the community, so that the views of the entire community can be represented.

Announcements about community meetings can also be sent in the form of an invitation to families. The invitation should list the times and locations of the various scheduled meetings and include a name and phone number to contact for more information. (See Example 2.)

Example 2

Community Meetings

Dear Family:

The Hilltop School District Health Education Curriculum Development Committee invites family and community members to comment on the plans for our new school health education curriculum. Your input will help the committee determine the content and teaching approaches for health education in the district. Four meetings have been scheduled.

Tuesday, September 13
South Side Middle School
*   Auditorium*
7:30 p.m.

Monday, September 19
Western Valley Elementary
*   School, Rm. 104*
7:30 p.m.

Wednesday, September 14
North Hill High School
*   Auditorium*
3:30 p.m.

Saturday, September 24
Hilltop School District Central
*   Administrative Office*
1:00 p.m.

Please attend the meeting that is most convenient for you. For more information, call 555-1234. We look forward to hearing from you.

Committee Responsibilities

To expand opportunities for family and community participation, committee members may be assigned roles or positions. A core committee could be responsible for decisions related to the entire curriculum, and task forces of additional members, including parents, could work on specific curriculum components. Task forces could be organized around content areas or grade levels.

Possible core committee members:

- curriculum coordinator, chair
- principal
- guidance coordinator
- health services coordinator
- senior high school health educator
- middle school health educator
- elementary education supervisor
- classroom teachers
- community members
- parents and other family members
- students

The committee is responsible for numerous tasks during the curriculum development process.

Curriculum development tasks:

- conducting a community needs assessment
- reviewing existing curriculum resources
- writing goals and objectives
- adopting, adapting or developing learning activities
- developing curriculum policies
- reviewing curriculum evaluation

Even though some of these tasks are the specific responsibility of professional staff members on the committee, community members can provide meaningful input and review.

Health Advisory Committees and Councils

Participation on a school health advisory committee or council provides another opportunity for family involvement in decision making about school health education. These groups often serve as steering committees on issues related to the comprehensive school health program. Health advisory committees and councils may address not only instruction but other areas of the comprehensive school health program, such as:

- health services
- the school environment
- guidance and counseling
- physical education
- food service

This type of participation may help family members gain a better sense of the various factors in and out of school that affect children's and adults' health. Working groups can be formed for all of the comprehensive health program areas addressed by the committee. This organizational structure presents an opportunity for even more family and community members to become involved.

Guidelines for this type of group are similar to those for curriculum development committees. Parents, family members and other community members are invited to participate in an open manner, and all members of the community have equal opportunity to contribute. Again, the composition of the committee should represent the entire community and all committee members should be engaged in meaningful tasks related to the group's overall mission.

Other Decision-Making Opportunities

Many other decision-making opportunities can be offered to family and community members. Additional committees may include staff members, parents and other community members working together on special projects, for example:

- reviewing audiovisual materials and other resources for the classroom
- reviewing complaints about instructional materials or teaching methods

In one large, inner-city elementary school, committees of parents and teachers were formed to interview and select candidates for both teacher and teacher aide positions. Before participating in interviews, parents were educated about qualities to look for in a good teacher or aide. This type of committee process was used to hire more than fifty teachers and aides.

The process has since become mandatory in each of the thirty elementary and secondary schools in the school district (Herman, 1993).

Health Education Programs for Family Members

Learning, both formal and informal, is a lifelong process. Health education programs for family and community members provide both knowledge and skills to help maintain and improve personal, family and community health.

Programs also help family and community members learn about the school health education program and develop skills to reinforce and enrich health learning at home and in the community. These programs may take place in a classroom setting or may be offered through more informal, independent approaches, such as a newsletter or a school-based center.

General Planning Guidelines

While sound educational principles are important regardless of the age or background of the participants, the following guidelines may be helpful when developing and implementing health education programs for adults.

1. Access
Plan programs for maximum access. Family members may be very interested in programs, but family and job responsibilities or lack of transportation may limit their participation. Programs can be designed to allow family members to participate in their homes or neighborhoods at different times during the day or evening.

2. Needs
Base program content on participants' needs. A needs assessment provides direction for planning programs that will meet the needs of the community.

3. Real World
Relate program content and activities to real-world experiences and situations. Focus on the realities of life in the community, offering knowledge and skills to help family members cope with those realities.

4. Diversity
Take advantage of participants' rich and diverse backgrounds. Such diversity will enrich the "texture" of the educational experience.

5. Development
Remember that adults are at different life stages and levels of development. Vary needs and expectations for different individuals. Written materials may need to be at varied reading levels, as well as in languages other than English.

6. Respect
Respect participants' values. Maintain a safe environment that promotes the free expression of varied personal opinions.

Types of Programs

Different types of programs meet different needs. Possibilities include:

- health information and education programs
- program awareness sessions
- course companion programs
- family centers

Example 3
Family Health Education Program

Dear Family,

Are you concerned about the amount of fatty foods your family eats? Would you like to learn how to prepare healthful snacks? Do you have questions about the new food labels?

The Hilltop School District will be offering a six-week nutrition class designed for parents and other adult family members. This free class will help you use the information on food labels to make healthy food choices and learn healthier ways to prepare foods for your family.

The class will meet weekly on Tuesday evenings from 8:00 p.m. to 9:30 p.m. in Room 210 at North Hill High School. For more information or to register for the class, please call 555-1234.

Health Information and Education Programs

Many adults need more health education. Direct educational programs on important topics, such as nutrition and food preparation, fitness, stress management, substance use and parenting, address this need.

These programs can be announced in several ways, including family letters. Letters should indicate the program's content and how it will benefit families. They should also include a number to call for more information or to register for the program. (See Example 3.)

Program Awareness Sessions

Program awareness sessions provide an overview of the specific health curriculum or program in a school. Families are often unaware of the goals, objectives, content and activities of health education courses.

Program awareness sessions are conducted by teachers to acquaint family members with the school health education program. They also help family members identify their roles in working with the student. Sessions may be held at the beginning of a course or at the beginning of individual course units.

Family letters can be used to invite attendance at these sessions. More people may be able to attend if several sessions are offered at a variety of dates, times and locations. (See Example 4.) If awareness sessions are held at the beginning of each course unit, the schedule should be drawn up and announced in advance. (See Example 5.)

The following guidelines can be used to develop and implement program awareness sessions:

1. **Adequate Notice**
Provide adequate notice to all parents. Inform parents of the date and time of the sessions. Identify the program and its purpose.

2. **Clear Agenda**
Organize the program with a clear agenda. Distribute copies of the agenda to all participants. (See Example 6.)

Example 4

Program Awareness Session

Dear Family,

Hilltop School District wants parents and other family members to be involved in their children's education. You are invited to learn more about your child's health education class. We are holding several awareness sessions that will include:

- *an overview of the course, including content, teaching methods and what the teacher will expect of students*

- *ways that parents and family members can be involved in the health education program*

- *time for open discussion and questions*

   The sessions will be held at the dates and times attached. You are welcome to come to any of these meetings. If you have any questions, please call the health education instructor at 555-1234.

Example 5

Schedule for Ongoing
Program Awareness Sessions

Topic:
Mental Health and Stress Management
Time/Date:
3:00 p.m. Wednesday, September 8
7:30 p.m. Thursday, September 9

Topic:
Nutrition and Fitness
Time/Date:
3:00 p.m. Wednesday, September 30
7:30 p.m. Thursday, October 1

Topic:
Alcohol, Tobacco and Other Drugs
Time/Date:
3:00 p.m. Wednesday, October 28
7:30 p.m. Thursday, October 29

Topic:
Sexuality
Time/Date:
3:00 p.m. Wednesday, November 18
7:30 p.m. Thursday, November 19

Topic:
Disease Prevention
Time/Date:
3:00 p.m. Wednesday, January 6
7:30 p.m. Thursday, January 7

All sessions will be held in Room 210 at North Hill High School.

Example 6

Awareness Session Agenda

11th Grade Health Education Program Awareness Session

Tuesday, September 15

8:00–9:30 p.m.

Agenda

Greeting/Introduction

Course Overview

Goals

Content

Teaching Methods

Student Expectations

Role of Family Members

Discussion

Closure

3. Course Goals

Present course goals and objectives, content and learning activities. You may need to explain that these sessions are not intended to provide time to discuss individual student progress.

4. Materials Display

Showcase students' work and instructional resources. Display examples of the work of all students if possible. Temporary displays can be posted in the hall outside the classroom or on bulletin boards in different areas of the school.

5. Open and Friendly

Be open and friendly. These sessions may be the first step toward a school/family partnership. Avoid the use of professional jargon.

6. Rationale for Involvement

Clearly explain the importance of family involvement. Describe some specific methods for family participation in students' education. Encourage parents to contact you with their questions and concerns and provide phone numbers and good times to call.

7. Time for Discussion

Always include time for dialogue. Be sure to schedule time at the end of the agenda for discussion and answering any questions parents may have.

Course Companion Programs

Course companion programs provide both direct health instruction and information about specific school health education curricula. These programs allow family members to learn about the same health topics their children are studying in health education class.

Course companion programs are particularly appropriate for middle schools and high schools, where health is offered as a separate course. Invitation letters to family members should include information about the content of the course, the time and location for the course and a contact number. (See Example 7.)

These programs are usually conducted by the classroom health education teacher. They include activities to help family members develop health knowledge and skills in the various topic areas covered in the school health education

Example 7

Course Companion Program

Dear Family:

You are invited to attend a special course for parents and other adults. The course will cover the topics that your child is studying in health class, but will focus on adult interests and concerns.

- *mental health*
- *stress management*
- *nutrition*
- *fitness*

- *tobacco, alcohol and other drugs*
- *sexuality*
- *disease prevention*
- *community health*

Each class session will include a brief discussion of what students are learning in the same topic area. Two classes will be held, one in the afternoon and one in the evening. The classes will be taught by Jennifer Nixon, North Hill High School Health Education Instructor.

If you have any questions or would like to sign up for one of the classes, please call 555-1234.

classroom. They also provide opportunities to discuss student reactions to the topic. Suggestions for dealing with the topic at home may also be offered. A typical agenda would include greetings, updates from the previous session, discussion of the current topic and what students are learning in class, and closure.

Family Centers

A family center is a room or available space devoted to offering health education materials for review by family members. Family and community members who are unable to make a commitment to a structured educational program or course may be interested in learning more about health and the school health education program on their own time. A family center helps meet their needs.

Using an open-door or walk-in policy, a center may be open to family members during the school day, as well as after school and in the evenings. It may provide materials and information on personal, family and community health topics. It can also offer information about the school health education program.

Suggested resources:

- books
- pamphlets
- audio cassettes
- videotapes
- assessment instruments
- computer programs
- district health education curriculum and resources
- examples of student assignments and projects
- monthly exhibits on specific health topics

Some of these resources, such as books and videotapes, could be made available to families on a loan basis. Others, such as pamphlets, could be distributed for visitors to keep.

An effective family center is more than just a reading room. It provides a place for family members to talk informally with school staff. Questionnaires, computer programs and other individualized learning activities will actively engage visitors. An information sheet can be used both to inform families about the center and invite them to visit. (See Example 8.)

The parent center at the Ellis School in Boston provides a model for future centers. This center focuses on the entire school curriculum, not just health education. It provides a "substantial, continuing and positive presence of family members in the school" (Davies, 1991). Parents report that it enables them to be more involved in and positive about their children's education.

Example 8
Family Health Education Center

Dear Family,

We invite you to visit the district's Family Health Education Center. This center helps families and other community members learn more about personal and community health. It also offers information about district health education programs.

Many materials are available for visitors to borrow, including:

- *books and videos*
- *audio cassettes*
- *pamphlets*
- *computer programs*

(continued...)

Example 8 *(continued)*

Family Health Education Center

Each month, the center features a special exhibit on a selected health topic. District health professionals are also available during certain hours to talk with visitors. The Family Health Education Center hours are 8:00 a.m. to 4:00 p.m. Monday through Friday, and 7:00 p.m. to 9:00 p.m. on Wednesday evenings.

The following people are there at the listed times to answer questions or talk with visitors:

District Health Education Coordinator
Tuesdays 3–4 p.m. and Thursdays 10–11 a.m.

District Health Services Director
Mondays 3–4 p.m. and Thursdays 9–10 a.m.

Community Medical Care Professional
Fridays 3–4 p.m.

At-Home Learning Activities for Families

Many parents and other family members may find it difficult to be involved in activities at the school site. Work schedules, childcare responsibilities, transportation difficulties and other circumstances may prevent individuals from being involved in school-based parent activities. Home-based student/family learning activities provide opportunities for parents who are unable to participate at school to be involved in their children's education. Activities that allow children and other family members to participate in learning at home offer the following benefits:

- reinforcement of topics and activities covered in the school health education class

- a forum for discussion of class topics that relate to family values

- improved family communication

- increased awareness of the school health education program

However, even with at-home activities, some students may have limited opportunities to participate with their family members. To avoid penalizing these students through grading or negative feedback, teachers can help them identify an adult or older youth to work with on the at-home activities, either at home, in the community or at another time during the school day. In some cases, the activity may need to be adapted or modified for the student's specific situation.

Developing At-Home Activities

At-home student/family learning activities have unlimited potential for involving family members and increasing the impact of education. Ideally, these activities will be developed in conjunction with a school district's health education curriculum. However, in practice, these activities are often developed to supplement an already existing program.

Considerations for developing and implementing activities:

- Family members may have limited time. They will not welcome time-consuming at-home activities every night of the school year.

- If all teachers in a school assign at-home family activities, interdisciplinary coordination will be needed.

- Clear instructions, including any answer sheets that may be needed, should be provided so family members completely understand the activity.

- Information should be presented in an attractive, professional manner.

Planning sheets or matrixes provide a format for examining the development of various activities in each of the content areas of comprehensive school health education. (See Example 9.)

Communicating with Families

Effective student/family activities include clear instructions for family members, as well as a description of the activity and its relationship to health education. Family members are encouraged to use these activities as springboards for family discussion of health topics. The most effective activities also include mechanisms for feedback from family members. When similar activities will be used throughout the course, an instruction sheet that describes each type of activity can be developed. (See Example 10.)

Individual activities can also be accompanied by family letters, or student memos at the high school level. Letters should clearly explain the assignment, including the student's responsibility and the family member's role. Any background materials adults might need to complete their aspect of the assignment should also be included. Letters should also include a phone number where family members can contact the teacher with any questions and an indication of the best times to call. Examples are included with each of the activities described below.

Example 9

Planning Sheet for Student/Family Learning Activities

Type of Family Activity

	Community Health	Consumer Health	Disease Prevention and Control	Environmental Health	Family Life	Injury Prevention and Safety	Mental and Emotional Health	Nutrition	Personal Health and Fitness	Substance Use Prevention
Review										
Collaborative Assignment										
Skills Practice										
Discussion Assignment										
Health Plan										
Calendar										
Home Activity Packet										

Example 10

At-Home Activities Instruction Sheet

Dear Family,

Your child's health education class this year will include many activities for students to complete with parents or other adult family members. The different types of activities you may see are listed here. Specific directions will be sent home with each activity as it is assigned.

- *Family Calendars*

- *Review Activities*

- *Family Collaborative Assignments*

- *Skills Practice*

- *Family Discussions*

- *Family Health Plans*

- *Home Activity Packets*

If you have any questions, please call me at 555-1234.

Types of Activities

Student/family learning activities involve a variety of approaches. These include:

- review activities
- collaborative assignments
- skills practice
- family discussion assignments
- family health plans
- family calendars
- home activity packets

Review Activities

Review activities are designed to reinforce classroom instruction. They usually involve a worksheet on which students respond either in writing or verbally. Family members then check the responses, based on an answer sheet provided for their use.

Examples of review activities:

- Second graders complete a worksheet that includes a drawing assignment and questions on bicycle safety. The worksheet is then reviewed with a family member. (See Example 11.)
- Middle school students respond to flash cards on fitness. The questions on the card are asked and checked by a family member, using answers printed on the back of the cards.
- High school students complete a crossword puzzle on nutrition. Their answers are checked and discussed by the student and a family member.
- High school students answer questions about a scenario related to a health topic. They discuss their responses with a family member. (See Example 12.)

Example 11
Elementary Review Activity

Dear Family,

Our class is studying bicycle safety. Your child has an activity sheet to complete to review the rules we have learned. To complete the activity, your child should draw pictures in the picture blocks that show these rules.

Under each picture block are questions for you to discuss with your child. Talking about these questions will help reinforce what your child learned in class. For your information, the pamphlet Bicycle Safety for Young Children, *from the Hilltop Health Department Safety Division, is included with this letter. You may want to read the pamphlet before going over the activity with your child.*

Thank you for being part of your child's health education. If you have any questions or need more information, please call me at 555-1234.

Example 12

High School Review Activity

To: 11th Grade Health Education Students

Your next assignment is based on scenarios that show teens and young adults making decisions about tobacco, alcohol and other drug use.

The first part of the assignment is to read the scenarios and answer several fact-related questions. Then please review your answers with a parent or another adult family member or friend. A copy of the **Drug Facts** *class handout is enclosed to help this person review your work. You also might want to discuss any issues brought up by the scenarios and listen to your family member's response to them.*

It is important for family members to learn information and skills together. I hope your family members will be involved in this activity. I can be reached at 555-1234.

Collaborative Assignments

Collaborative assignments involve work done cooperatively with other family members. Unlike review assignments, students and family members work together to complete collaborative assignments. These assignments may involve work that can be completed in the home or assignments outside the home setting.

Examples of collaborative assignments:

- Elementary school students and family members shop together for supplies for a family first-aid kit.

- Middle school students and family members complete a questionnaire on family health history. (See Example 13.)

- High school students and family members read a magazine or newspaper article on health care and together answer a series of questions based on the article.

Skills Practice

Skills learned in health education classes are often used in real-life settings outside of school. Skills practice with family members provides a real-world laboratory in which students and family members can reinforce healthy behaviors.

Generic skills can be taught across all health education content areas. Fetro (1992) has identified decision making, communication, stress management and goal setting as generic skills. Other skills may be topic specific, such as reading nutrition labels, administering CPR, using a condom, or planning a family exercise program.

Five steps for promoting skills development:

1. Introduce the skill.
2. Present steps for developing the skill.
3. Model the skill.
4. Practice and rehearse the skill.
5. Provide feedback and reinforcement.

The home and community provide many opportunities to model and practice skills, as well as ways to provide feedback and reinforcement.

Example 13

Middle School Collaborative Assignment

Dear Family,

Thank you for your help with your child's assignments. Parents and other family members are a great help in reviewing and reinforcing what students learn in class.

The first assignment in our unit on disease prevention is a family collaborative assignment. Students and family members work together on the activity.

Your child has a family health history questionnaire. You may not be able to answer all the questions. But please complete those that you can answer and are comfortable responding to.

Next week I will be sending home a packet of information for your family about disease prevention. Please call if you have any questions or need more information. I can be reached at 555-1234.

Examples of skills practice activities:

- First grade students and family members walk together through the school playground or to the bus stop, discussing and demonstrating pertinent safety rules.

- Fourth grade students discuss with family members situations in which they had to resist pressure. After discussing personal experiences, they discuss possible responses to situations in which resistance skills are needed.

- Before a family walk, seventh grade students and family members calculate their target heart rates.

- During a nutrition unit, tenth grade students work with family members, using notes from class, to prepare a typical family meal, using food preparation methods that lower the fat and sodium content. (See Example 14.)

Family Discussion Assignments

Many topics in health education relate to family values. Structured family discussions allow students to discuss values-related issues with family members.

Examples of family discussion assignments:

- After reading aloud a short story from a second grade assignment, family members discuss and evaluate the main character's decisions.

- After completing a worksheet related to tobacco, alcohol and other drug use decisions, middle school students share and discuss their responses with family members. (See Example 15.)

- After watching a television show on teen sexuality, middle or high school students and family members complete a worksheet containing discussion questions on issues covered in the program.

- In class, high school students work in cooperative learning groups to develop a plan for local, state or national government to address the HIV epidemic. Once the plan is developed, students present it to family members for discussion.

Example 14
High School Skills Practice

Dear Family:

As part of our unit on nutrition, I would like students to work with family members to prepare a typical family meal using food preparation methods that help lower the fat and sodium content of the meal. Your son or daughter has a fact sheet with tips on how to prepare meals that are lower in fat and sodium.

Your son or daughter also has an activity sheet to complete after preparing the meal. If your family is already cooking with less fat and sodium, you might want to try preparing something new rather than a typical family meal. Another assignment is available for students who are unable to prepare a meal.

I appreciate your efforts to be involved in your son or daughter's health education. Please contact me at 555-1234 if you need further information.

Example 15

Middle School Family Discussion Assignment

Dear Family,

Our next family assignment has been designed to help promote family discussions about tobacco, alcohol and other drugs. Please respond to the short scenarios described on your child's assignment sheet. These scenarios focus on making decisions about drug use. Your discussion might include facts, alternatives, consequences, and personal and family values.

*Students have a **Drug Fact Sheet** and a **Decision-Making Model** information sheet to use in this activity. They also have a **Student Reaction Sheet** to complete, as well as an optional **Family Reaction Sheet**.*

Please feel free to contact me at 555-1234 if you have any questions.

Family Health Plans

Family health plans provide students and family members an opportunity to identify and improve selected health behaviors. Family plans can be developed for each unit in the health education curriculum or for selected units. Each plan should be based on knowledge and skills developed by students in class. The activity may include a sheet on which families can record their reactions to the activity.

Examples of family health plans:

- Elementary students and family members develop a plan to select a book related to each health unit and read it together. The reading is scheduled on a regular basis.

- Middle school student and family members participate twice a week in physical activity, such as a family bike outing, a family walk or a family volleyball game. (See Example 16.)

- High school students and family members work together on a regular basis to improve family nutrition. Activities may include family preparation of one nutritious meal per week or a meal at a favorite family restaurant in which low-fat dishes are chosen.

Family Calendars

Family calendars can be used to promote daily family discussion of topics covered in class. This discussion is meant to be quick (less than five minutes) and involve as many family members as possible. Calendars can be developed for each topic covered during the health education course. Families can be encouraged to display calendars in a prominent place, such as the refrigerator door or family bulletin board. (See Example 17.)

Home Activity Packets

Home activity packets provide a collection of activities and resources for students to take home and review with family members. They focus on a specific health education topic and include materials that can engage family members on both an individual and group basis.

Example 16

Middle School Family Health Plan

Our family agrees to do the following physical activity twice a week:

Activity: *8-mile family bike ride*

Times: *Tuesday and Friday evenings*

Signed:

Record time, distance or any other comments about the activity.

	Day	Time/Distance	Day	Time/Distance	Comments
Week 1					
Week 2					
Week 3					
Week 4					
Week 5					
Week 6					
Week 7					
Week 8					

Family Reactions

In the space below, family members can write a brief reaction to the plan. Each family member should sign her or his name.

Example 17

Family Calendar

Topic: Nutrition

	Week 1		**Week 2**
Day 1	What are your family's favorite food sources of Vitamins A and C? Do family members have daily sources of Vitamins A and C?	**Day 6**	Schedule a time during the next week to plan a healthy family snack. Discuss the food items you will need.
Day 2	Find a food item in the kitchen that is a complex carbohydrate. Discuss favorite ways to eat this food.	**Day 7**	Identify foods that family members enjoy that should be eaten in moderation.
Day 3	What are your family's favorite high-fiber foods? How often do family members eat these foods?	**Day 8**	Identify your family's favorite fast-food restaurant. How can foods at the restaurant be ordered to make them more nutritious?
Day 4	Review a food label from a food in your kitchen. Is it a good source of any nutrients? Is it high in fat, sodium or sugar?	**Day 9**	Discuss a television advertisement for a food item. What claims are the advertisers making to convince you to buy the food?
Day 5	Discuss family snacking habits. Which snacks are healthy snacks?	**Day 10**	Are there situations in which family members feel pressured to eat less nutritious foods? Discuss different ways to respond.

Packets may be packaged in a briefcase, pencil box, knapsack or other portable container. Most are used on a loan basis and returned to the school, although if multiple copies exist, materials can be given to families. A list of included materials should be developed for each type of packet, and an inventory should be taken when the packets are returned to school.

Ideally, each student would have an activity packet for the entire unit. Depending on the packet contents, however, this might be too costly. In this case, a limited number of packets can be developed for each instructional unit and families can take turns using them.

Possible resources for activity packets:

- a videotape for family viewing and discussion
- a case study related to the unit topic
- a list of ideas for family projects
- a crossword puzzle for individual or family completion
- related magazine or newspaper articles
- an audiotape for family listening and discussion
- instructions for a family health skill, such as meal preparation or first-aid techniques
- ideas for family health plans
- flashcards for content review
- a game related to the topic
- a journal or log in which family members can write their reactions to the packet activities or suggestions for other activities

Organization of such packets requires time and effort. Teachers may want to start by developing a limited number of packets with a few materials for one instructional unit. Additional materials and packets can be added over time. (See Example 18.)

Example 18
Home Activity Packet

Dear Family,

You have just received, for a loan period of five days, the Cardiovascular Health Home Activity Packet. A laminated card lists all of the materials that should be in the packet.

The packet includes a videotape, Steps to Cardiovascular Health; *view this individually or as a group. The pamphlets are yours to keep. You may also keep copies of the* **Family Heart Health Assessment** *and the* **Cardiovascular Health Crossword Puzzle**.

I hope that this packet adds to your family's health awareness. Please have each family member complete the **Participant Journal** and return the packet by November 10.

Please call me at 555-1234 if you have any questions. Thank you.

Other Ways to Reach Families

Some families may be harder to reach than others. In communities where significant obstacles make it difficult for many family members to access the school site, additional efforts may be needed. Two effective strategies are neighborhood programs, which bring the programs to the families, and newsletters, which provide a convenient source of information.

Providing Neighborhood Programs

Participating in activities at the school site may sometimes be difficult or impossible, even when family members are very interested in the program. Bringing programs to the neighborhoods served by the school can increase family and community involvement. Health information and education programs, program awareness sessions, course companion programs and even family centers can be located in neighborhoods.

Creativity is often the key in bringing programs to neighborhoods. Audrey Sullivan, principal at Hans Christian Andersen Elementary School in Rockledge, Florida, described plans for a "whistle-stop" tour on one of her school district's inservice days. Teachers ride the school bus to different neighborhoods and stop at various locations to meet with family members and distribute information ("The Parent Factor," 1991).

Similar efforts could be developed for school health programs. Letters, similar to those used for other family involvement programs, can inform and invite families to these events. (See Example 19.)

Using Newsletters for Outreach

Newsletters can serve as an educational tool to reach family members. They can provide information about personal, family and community health, and school health education programs. Newsletters may be sent home with students, mailed to parents or made available to community members in different locations throughout the district.

Example 19

Neighborhood Awareness Programs

Dear Family or Community Member:

The Hilltop School District will be holding a series of neighborhood health education awareness programs. These programs can help parents and other community members learn more about our school health education program.

The initial meetings will cover:

- *content of the school health education program*
- *teaching techniques*
- *expectations for students*
- *ways that parents and other family members can be involved*

Times, dates and locations for our first meetings are attached. We hope you will be able to attend at least one. If you have any questions, please call 555-1234.

Teachers or other professional staff can develop a newsletter, or students can assume all or part of the responsibility. Students might work on a newsletter as part of a class assignment or as part of an extracurricular activity, such as a health or journalism club. The Cajon Family/School Partnership in California provided parents and students with after-school workshops on desktop publishing, after which parents and students worked together to produce student publications ("The FIRST Grants," 1991).

4

Assessing and Improving Family Involvement

*Family-based programs theoretically have enormous poten-
tial because the family provides the most potent role models
for health education, enabling change by reducing barriers and by appropriate reinforcements.*

—Cheryl Perry

The most effective family involvement activities result from a systematic analysis of existing activities and needs, followed by precise planning to develop an effective action approach. Comprehensive assessment and planning activities promote meaningful involvement in health education for family and other community members. They also help improve health education programs for students and the health of both students and family members.

An assessment process will help examine the school or district's commitment to family involvement as well as the current level of family involvement in the district and schools. The assessment then can serve as the basis for planning for improved family and community involvement.

Planning the Assessment

The assessment process begins with a staff awareness meeting—a discussion of the family involvement efforts in which all school or district staff should be included. The discussion can cover the rationale for parent and family involvement, as well as different opportunities for such involvement.

This initial meeting provides a forum for open discussion of staff ideas and concerns about the family involvement process, as well as the strategies currently being used to involve parents and family members. It should conclude with a clear presentation of the school district's commitment to parent and family involvement, including the provision of inservice training for staff and time for teacher planning of involvement activities.

After the staff awareness meeting, a family involvement assessment and planning committee can be formed. Likely members of this committee include administrators, teachers, parents and other family members, community members and students. This committee is responsible for conducting the assessment, developing a report on the results, and developing an action plan for improving family involvement. (See Figure 3.)

Figure 3
Assessment and Planning Process

Step 1: Hold staff awareness meeting.
Step 2: Form assessment committee.
Step 3: Conduct assessment.

- Examine commitment to family involvement.

- Interview administrators.

- Interview teachers.

- Interview parents and other family members.

- Interview students.

Step 4: Develop assessment report.
Step 5: Present report to appropriate level of school district administration.
Step 6: Conduct action planning.

- List needs.

- Develop plan.

Step 7: Present action plan to appropriate level of school district administration.

As with other decision-making committees that involve family and community members, committee membership needs to reflect the different family cultures in the community. Teachers will represent those responsible for teaching health education, and several students can be chosen to represent the middle and high school grades.

Conducting the Assessment

The assessment begins after the committee is formed. An effective assessment process will evaluate district and school efforts in the following areas:

- school district commitment
- involvement of family and other community members in decision making
- education programs for family and other community members
- at-home student/family learning activities

The information acquired in the assessment will be used to provide a profile of the district's current efforts in family involvement. Inquiries, therefore, should focus on "what is" rather than "what could be" or "what should be." Interviews can be assigned to individual committee members, who can then report back to the committee.

The *Family Involvement Assessment Inventory* can be used as a framework for the assessment. (See Appendix B.) All items in the inventory are important. The following steps provide a guide to conducting the review.

Assessment Inventory Steps

1. Examine Commitment to Family Involvement
Review the school or district's philosophy, policy and mission statement for evidence of emphasis on the importance of family involvement.

2. Interview Administrators

Appropriate administrators should be interviewed regarding the following components:

- nature of messages sent to families

- staff attitudes toward families

- commitment to inservice training

- commitment to teacher planning time for family involvement

- evaluation of family involvement efforts

- family involvement in decision making

- education programs for families

3. Interview Teachers

Health education teachers or their representatives should be interviewed regarding the following components:

- nature of messages sent to families

- staff attitudes toward families

- commitment to inservice training

- commitment to teacher planning time for family involvement

- evaluation of family involvement efforts

- involvement in decision making

- education programs for parents

- at-home student/family learning activities

4. Interview Parents and Other Family Members

A sample of family members who represent all family cultures in the community should be interviewed regarding the following components:

- nature of messages sent to families

- staff attitudes toward families

- involvement in decision making

- education programs for families
- at-home student/family learning activities

5. Interview Students
Students who represent all segments of the student body should be interviewed regarding the following components:

- staff attitudes toward families
- at-home student/family learning activities

As information is gathered, findings can be compiled on a master copy of the assessment. (See Appendix B.) When all interviews have been completed, the entire committee meets to hear the results. This information can then be compiled into a final version of the assessment inventory, with all items appropriately marked and final comments included.

The final version of the assessment inventory can then be presented to the appropriate level of the school district administration. This body may be the school board, administrative team, curriculum coordinator or other appropriate individual or group.

After reviewing the assessment, the district can evaluate its commitment to the improvement of family involvement based on the report. Once the district commitment is determined, the committee is ready to move to the action planning phase.

Action Planning

Action planning begins with a committee review of the final assessment inventory report. The committee then lists, in priority order, the needs identified in the report. (See Figure 4 for an example.) Most of the needs will probably relate to assessment items that were judged to be in the categories "Needs Improvement" or "Does Not Exist."

Once the needs have been listed for each section, the committee can identify those that can be addressed in the action plan, based on the school district's expressed commitment and available resources. Action plan goals will be based on the four areas examined by the assessment inventory. (See Appendix C.)

Figure 4

Family Involvement Needs

(Needs listed in priority order.)

1. Revise mission statement.

2. Provide staff training.

3. Increase parental involvement in decision making.

4. Develop selected education program for parents and family members.

5. Add all seven types of at-home student/family learning activities to curriculum.

Specific objectives can be developed for each goal or for those goals determined to be important for the school or district. Initially, only small steps may be possible to address some needs.

If possible, all needs should be addressed in some way, even if only by investigating sources of support to address a need in the future. For example, a district may see no possibility to provide space for a family center in the near future due to overcrowded school buildings. Rather than not addressing the need at all, a first step might be for the committee to write a letter to the district school board and school task force on expansion (or a similar group) describing the benefits of a family center and the space that would be required. Such action would at least support the need for extra space.

Another possible small step might be the addition of a mini-collection of health materials in an area of the school frequented by visitors. While certainly not the equivalent of a family center, such a collection can be a positive first step.

The objectives developed to address the identified needs should be actions that can be easily assessed or measured for attainment. Each objective should contribute to the attainment of the goal for that section of the action plan. Tasks related to each objective are those activities that need to be undertaken to accomplish the objective. (See Figure 5 for an example.) If more precision in planning is desired, responsibility for completion of the tasks can be assigned to specific individuals along with completion dates.

In order that family involvement activities have the most impact, a systematic analysis of existing activities and needs must be carried out. The step by step process and assessment inventory presented in this chapter should provide the basis for this endeavor. The action planning format should provide a precise pathway for the development of a meaningful action approach. Readers who follow this assessment and action planning process should rely on the earlier chapters in this book for background and direction. Quality, comprehensive assessment, planning, and action should lead to more meaningful involvement in health education for parents and family members, improved health education programs for students, and hopefully better health for students and family members.

Figure 5

Action Plan Example

Goal: To improve the district's commitment to family involvement in school health education.

Objective 1:

Revise school mission statement to reflect the importance of parents as partners in education.

Tasks:

1a. Form committee to review mission statement and revise. (Responsibility: assistant superintendent and parent volunteer coordinator.)
1b. Convene committee and work on revision. (Responsibility: committee chair.)

Objective 2:

Improve health education instructional staff's knowledge and skills related to family involvement.

Tasks:

2a. Develop a compilation of relevant literature in parent involvement for staff review. (Responsibility: curriculum coordinator and health education department chair.)
2b. Plan and conduct staff development program for instructional staff. (Responsibility: curriculum coordinator and health education department chair.)

5

Preparing Teachers for Family Involvement

Few teacher education institutions prepare teachers to communicate with parents, even though parent involvement has been shown to have positive effects on children's achievement.

—Bermudez and Padron

Recent national education goals emphasize the importance of training teachers for family involvement. One of the goals in the *Goals 2000: Educate America Act* is for increased parent participation in schools. Another of the goals provides further impetus for inservice training: Teachers will have the professional development they need to help students reach the other goals.

The ability to engage family members as partners in education is not an inherent skill. However, this area of teacher preparation has received little attention. A survey of 575 teacher educators found that only 4 percent of their programs offered a complete course on the topic of parent/teacher relations and 15 percent offered part of a course, while 37 percent reported that a required course was needed (Chavkin and Williams, 1988). Teacher training needs have two aspects:

- Inservice training for employed teachers
- Preservice training for student teachers

Preservice training in health education related to family involvement is justified by several competencies and sub-competencies in the Responsibilities and Competencies for Entry Level Health Educators as identified by the National Task Force on the Preparation and Practice of Health Educators (Appendix D). These competencies provide the framework for National Committee for the Accreditation of Teacher Education Programs approval of health education professional preparation programs.

Key Components of Training

Important components of comprehensive professional preparation programs in family involvement, at both the inservice and preservice levels, include the following.

1. Information

Provide information about the potential of family involvement. Research shows the positive effects of family involvement in education. Data also show that parents and other family members are interested and willing to be involved in their children's education.

2. Diversity

Offer insights into family diversity. All school staff need to appreciate the differences among families. Students come to school with varied cultural, ethnic, religious and socioeconomic experiences. This diversity should be viewed as a richness that contributes positively to the uniqueness of each school site.

3. Skills

Teach skills for both verbal and written communication with family members. Some family members may be reluctant to be involved with the school because of perceived barriers to communication. The best communication uses clear, simple language and avoids professional jargon. In many districts, some families will need both written and verbal communication in languages other than English. All communication should openly encourage parents and other family members to participate as partners with school staff in their children's education.

4. Roles

Examine decision-making roles for parents and other family members. Family members can participate in decision making related to many aspects of the school program, including curriculum development, school health advisory committees and materials review committees.

5. Programs

Provide information about education programs targeted to families. Several types of education programs can be developed for family members and conducted by the school health educator. Possible programs include health education sessions, program awareness sessions, course companion programs, family centers, neighborhood programs and newsletters.

6. Practice

Offer practice in developing and facilitating at-home learning activities. One of the most important components of professional preparation for family involvement is activities that help participants learn to develop at-home student/family learning activities, such as review activities, collaborative assignments, skills practice, discussion assignments, health plans, calendars and activity packets.

A Model for Inservice Training

Inservice training has special considerations. For many teachers, the idea of involving parents and other family members as partners in the instructional program may appear an almost impossible task. Teachers need opportunities to address their concerns about involving family members. One strategy is to phase in family involvement efforts gradually, allowing teachers adequate time to prepare and implement involvement activities. Training should be an ongoing process that includes time for debriefing initial implementation efforts.

Training Outline

A one-day (six-hour) inservice training program could include the following activities. (See Figure 6 for a sample agenda.)

Rationale for Family Involvement

Begin the activity by brainstorming responses to the question "Why should we involve parents and other family members in health education?" List the responses on the board or on an overhead transparency. Be sure to include the following:

- Parents influence behavior that students practice now and in the future.
- Parents want to be involved in their children's education.
- Families can become educated about health.
- Families can provide reinforcement to classroom instruction.
- Parents present a family perspective on sensitive topics.
- Families can learn about school health education and become program supporters.
- Family involvement has a positive impact on student learning.

Figure 6

One-Day Inservice Training on Family Involvement

Agenda

8:30–8:40	Greeting/Overview of Agenda
8:40–9:00	Introductory Activity
9:00–9:30	Rationale for Family Involvement
9:30–9:45	Types of Family Involvement
9:45–10:30	Challenges and Barriers
10:30–10:45	Break
10:45–11:00	The School District's Responsibility
11:00–11:30	Family Cultures
11:30–12:00	Family Members as Decision Makers
12:00–1:00	Lunch
1:00–1:30	Educational Programs for Family Members
1:30–3:00	Development of At-Home Learning Activities
3:00–3:20	Action Planning Process
3:20–3:30	Closure

Introductory Activity

Show participants various quotes, displayed on an overhead projector, or provide a handout with the quotes. (See Figure 7.) Ask participants to move around the room and find one person (preferably someone whom they don't know or haven't talked with recently) with whom to discuss their response to the first quote and its relationship to health education. After a few minutes, direct participants to move to another person and discuss the second quote. Continue in this manner until all quotes have been discussed. Then discuss responses to the quotes with the whole group.

Figure 7
Quotes to Spark Discussion

Parent/Child Interaction

The interaction between parents and children may well be the most important key to lasting, long-term improvements in the overall health status of this country.

—*James O. Mason*

Educating a Child

The whole village educates the child.

—*African Proverb*

Family-Based Programs

Family-based programs theoretically have enormous potential because the family provides the most potent role models for health education, enabling change by reducing barriers and by appropriate reinforcements.

—*Cheryl Perry*

The Context for Health Education

Health education occurs in the context of family, community, religious, and media messages concerning health.

—*Maurice Elias*

Communicating with Parents

Few teacher education institutions prepare teachers to communicate with parents, even though parent involvement has been shown to have positive effects on children's achievement.

—*Bermudez and Padron*

Types of Family Involvement

Present the general categories of family involvement:

- involvement of family members in decision making
- educational programs directed toward family members
- at-home student/family learning activities

Challenges and Barriers

In small groups, have participants identify what they see as challenges or barriers to family involvement. Have a recorder from each group report the challenges and barriers identified by that group. Address concerns. (See Figure 8 for some examples.)

The School District's Responsibility

The sample policy in Appendix A can provide a framework for this activity. If the participants are all from the same school district, the district's actual commitment or policy can be reviewed or possible actions discussed with participants. If the participants are from different districts, general ideas about how a district can make a commitment to family involvement can be presented.

Family Cultures

Present and discuss various family cultures. Topics addressed will be determined somewhat by the cultures represented in the participants' school district(s).

Family Members as Decision Makers

Present a list of possible roles that family members can play in educational decision making, including the following:

- curriculum development committees
- health advisory committees and councils
- resource review committees

Figure 8

Addressing Concerns About Family Involvement

Some students have no support at home and do not live in traditional family structures.

Research indicates that most parents, even those in what would be considered nontraditional family structures, want to be involved in their children's education. In some situations, other available adults (school staff, community leaders, etc.) can be used as substitutes for family members.

All parents or families will not be involved.

True, but with structured efforts the number of parents and family members involved will increase. Schools must reach out to involve as many parents as possible. Students should not be penalized in any way if their parents are not involved.

How will I find the time to plan and be involved in such programs?

Planning time is essential for parent and family involvement activities. With limited planning time, efforts to increase parent involvement may have to start out on a small scale and gradually increase over time. The school district commitment to family involvement must include providing time for teacher preparation and planning.

What about the district administration? Will they support us?

Administrative support is absolutely necessary. School districts should develop a family involvement policy and/or strategic plan that specifically identifies the role of the school administration relative to program support.

Many of my student's parents speak a different language. How can I communicate with them?

For in-person meetings with parents, if necessary, a translator should be available. Written materials should be written in English and other appropriate languages. Schools can also form advisory committees to address ways of improving communication.

- controversial issues review committees
- interview/selection teams or committees

Educational Programs for Family Members

List different types of educational programs for family members. These include:
- health information and education programs
- program awareness sessions
- course companion programs
- family centers
- neighborhood programs
- newsletters

Development of At-Home Learning Activities

This topic is a critical component of the session. Give participants the opportunity to spend time developing at least one student/family at-home activity, either working individually or in groups. Teachers of the same grade level are often more creative and productive working in groups. Activities should be based on the actual curriculum that participants use in their teaching.

Prior to developing the at-home activities, discuss the various types of activities available.

- review activities
- collaborative assignments
- skills practice
- family discussion assignments
- family health plans
- family calendars
- home activity packets

Provide time for participants to share and discuss the activities they have developed.

Action Planning Process

This segment provides participants time to develop a plan to use the information and skills they have acquired. Typically, action plans include goals, objectives, tasks and timelines. Possible action plan goals include:

• assessing current family involvement efforts in the district's program

• sharing information with other staff members in the district

• infusing family involvement into the existing health education curriculum

• developing an educational program for family members

If more than one day can be allotted to the training, some needs assessment could be conducted before a detailed action plan is developed. The purpose of action planning during a one-day session is to develop a plan for teachers to take the next step for improved family involvement. This next step may involve conducting a more extensive needs assessment.

Closure

At the end of the training, provide time for participants to offer feedback about the training to the facilitator. Feedback can be both verbal and written. During this time, participants can also be given a final chance to ask any questions or address any additional barriers they perceive or concerns they might have.

Preservice Training Considerations

Faculty members in health education professional preparation programs can identify opportunities for students to develop the knowledge and skills needed to facilitate family involvement activities before they enter the classroom.

Such training is justified by several of the competencies and subcompetencies included in the *Responsibilities and Competencies for Entry-Level Health Educators* identified by the National Task Force on the Preparation and Practice of Health Educators, which provide the framework for approval of health education professional preparation programs. (Appendix D lists those competencies that relate to family and community involvement.)

The following five actions by college and university faculty could lead to more emphasis on preparing students to involve families in school health education:

1. Staff Development
Provide staff development programs for current college/university faculty members to develop the background necessary to incorporate family involvement concepts and activities into their classes.

2. Existing Classes
Identify topics and activities in existing classes that could be expanded to address family involvement, such as adding a family involvement activity to the lessons students are to develop in a methods course.

3. New Course
Develop a course or workshop that focuses on family involvement, either through the health education department or as a collaborative effort with another department, such as education or family studies.

4. Student Research
Identify student research opportunities related to family involvement, such as surveys of teacher needs or concerns related to involving families, evaluation of current family involvement efforts, or willingness of parents to be involved.

5. Student Teachers
Emphasize family involvement during the student teaching experience.

Family Involvement Activities for Preservice

A variety of activities can be used to help college students in professional preparation programs develop knowledge and skills to conduct family involvement activities. (*Note:* The term *student(s),* when used in the following descriptions, refers to college students in professional programs, not students in the K-12 classroom.)

Introductory Letter for a Health Education Course or Unit

Letters are often sent home to provide parents and other family members with an overview of their children's classes. Students can write an introductory letter to parents. The letter would present an overview of the course, including topic areas, importance of family involvement, nature of homework assignments, and any other relevant information. Similar letters can be developed for specific units in a health education course.

Parental Meeting Simulation

Most school districts conduct "Open House" or "Back to School" programs for parents at the beginning of the school year. Such programs provide a valuable opportunity to present information about classes. Working individually or in groups, students develop both a letter for parents regarding such a program and an agenda for the presentation. One or several students can conduct the presentation, with other students acting as attending parents and family members.

At-Home Student/Family Learning Activities

Students in professional programs often develop lesson plans and units as part of their class requirements. An additional component of these assignments could be to develop corresponding at-home student/family learning activities. After such activities have been developed, they can be presented in class to be reviewed by and shared with other students.

Newsletters

This activity could also be implemented in conjunction with student development of units or lesson plans. Students could create a newsletter that informs parents about the content of the unit and provides suggestions for reinforcing the instructional focus of the unit at home. Additional current health information for parents can also be included.

Family Calendars

A family calendar can be developed in conjunction with a learning unit. For each lesson in the unit, students could develop a corresponding quick family activity. These activities would then be incorporated into a calendar that could be sent home to parents. Ideally, the calendars would be included as part of either the introductory letter or a unit newsletter.

Parent Conference Simulation

Conferences with parents are an important activity for all teachers. To simulate a conference, the university instructor could develop profiles of several hypothetical children and/or youth. Working in pairs, one student would play the teacher, using one of the profiles for the conference. The other student would play an adult family member. After the simulated conference is completed, partners switch roles and use a different profile. After all pairs have completed their simulated conferences, the activity is processed by the entire group.

Literature, Television and Movies

Many children's books, television programs and movies either address health topics or relate to concepts covered in health education. Since reading or viewing generally occurs at home, literature, television and film (video) present opportunities for family involvement activities.

For this activity, students select a television program, book or movie for use as a family involvement activity. They then develop a description of an assignment that could be sent home to parents. The description should include a summary of the book, movie or program, an idea of how the source is related to the topic being covered in health education and directions for the assignment. This activity could also be directly related to the learning units developed by students.

Family/Community Culture

Many students have little opportunity to interact on an adult level with family and other community members in regard to education and health. The culture of preservice students in college involves interests, priorities and communication styles that are very different from many family and community cultures. However, upon graduation, new teachers must be prepared to interact productively with the family members of the children in their classrooms.

To prepare students for this interaction, opportunities for observing and interacting with the community must be provided, such as attending PTA and school board meetings, participating in other community events and meetings, and interviewing parents about their health education interests and concerns. Students can then write a summary of the experience and their reactions to it and discuss the results as a class.

Student Teaching

For students in professional preparation programs in education, the student-teaching experience provides the culmination of undergraduate training. This experience also should provide an opportunity to develop skills in involving family members in school health education.

Student teachers can be expected to develop family involvement activities for lessons and units they develop and teach. In addition, student teachers can be asked to participate in parent/teacher conferences and attend other events that will help them develop communication skills and become familiar with family cultures. These experiences should be reviewed with student teaching supervisors, just as other aspects of student teaching are.

Appendix A

Sample Family Involvement Policy

The (state/district/school board) recognizes that a child's education is a responsibility shared by the school and the family. Education professionals and families must work as knowledgeable partners in order to educate all students to their greatest capacity. To this end, the Board supports the development, implementation and regular evaluation of a family involvement policy and program that involves all parents and families at all grade levels in a variety of roles.

Although families are diverse in culture and language, they share the school's commitment to the educational success of their children.

Each school, in collaboration with parents and families, shall establish and develop programs and practices that enhance family involvement and address the specific needs of students and families. The policy and program will be comprehensive and coordinated and will include, but not be limited to, the following efforts:

- Include parents and families as leaders and decision makers in school issues and programs.

- Promote clear, two-way communication between school and family about instructional programs and children's progress.

- Assist parents, families and guardians in developing parenting skills and acquiring techniques to support their children's learning.

- Involve parents and family members, where appropriate, in instructional and support roles at the school.

- Provide access to and coordinate community and support services for children and families.

- Identify and reduce barriers to family involvement.

- Provide professional development for teachers and staff on ways to work effectively with parents and families.

- Provide a written copy of the policy for each parent and/or family and post the policy in the school.

These forms of involvement, which can overlap, require a coordinated schoolwide and communitywide effort.

Source: The National PTA, Chicago, Illinois. This policy is based, in part, on the *Parent Involvement Policy* adopted in 1989 by the California State Board of Education.

Appendix B

Family Involvement Assessment Inventory

S = Satisfactory   **N** = Needs Improvement   **D** = Does Not Exist

I. School District Commitment

	S	N	D

A. A clear statement exists in the school philosophy or mission statement of the importance of including family and other community members as partners in education.
Comments:

B. Numerous clear messages are sent to families regarding their possible roles and responsibilities as partners.
Comments:

C. Staff members acknowledge and validate the worth and potential positive influence of all individuals from all family structures and situations.
Comments:

                                                                    S N D

D. Teachers and other staff members are provided with the inservice   □ □ □
training needed to develop and implement parent involvement efforts.
Comments:

E. Teachers and other staff members have adequate time to develop,   □ □ □
implement and evaluate parent involvement activities.
Comments:

F. All aspects of the school district family involvement program are   □ □ □
evaluated.
Comments:

II. Involvement of Family Members in Decision Making   **S N D**
A. Family and community members are involved in decision-making   □ □ □
processes in education.
Comments:

Note: If family involvement in decision making is nonexistent, do
not answer **B** or **C**. Move directly to Part III.

B. All family members in all segments of the community have equal   □ □ □
access to recruiting announcements for participation in curriculum
development.
Comments:

	S	N	D

C. All segments of the community are represented in decision-making efforts. □ □ □
Comments:

III. Education Programs for Families

A. The following education programs are offered for family members.

	S	N	D
1. Health information and education sessions	□	□	□
2. Program awareness sessions	□	□	□
3. Course companion programs	□	□	□
4. Family centers	□	□	□
5. Neighborhood projects	□	□	□
6. Newsletters	□	□	□

Comments:

IV. At-Home Student/Family Learning Activities

A. At-home student/family learning activities are offered by the district. □ □ □

Note: If activities are nonexistent, do not answer **B.** You have completed the inventory.

B. The following types of at-home student/family activities are included as part of the curriculum.

	S	N	D
• Review activities	□	□	□
• Collaborative assignments	□	□	□
• Skills practice	□	□	□
• Family discussion assignments	□	□	□
• Family health plans	□	□	□
• Family calendars	□	□	□
• Home activity packets	□	□	□

Comments:

Appendix C

Family Involvement Action Plan

I. School District Commitment

Goal: To improve the district's commitment to family involvement in school health education.

Objective:

Tasks:

Objective:

Tasks:

II. Involvement of Family Members in Decision Making

Goal: To increase involvement of family and community members in decision making in the district.

Objective:

Tasks:

Objective:

Tasks:

III. Education Programs for Families

Goal: To improve education programs for family and community members in the district.

Objective:

Tasks:

Objective:

Tasks:

IV. At-Home Student/Family Learning Activities

Goal: To improve at-home student/family learning activities for students and family members in the district.

Objective:

Tasks:

Objective:

Tasks:

Appendix D

Competencies and Subcompetencies Related to Family Involvement

Note: This appendix lists only those competencies
that relate to family involvement.

Responsibility I—Assessing Individual and Community Needs for Health Education

Competency A: Obtain health-related data about social and cultural environments, growth and development factors, needs and interests.

Competency B: Distinguish between behaviors that foster, and those that hinder, well-being.

Subcompetencies: (1) Investigate physical, social, emotional and intellectual factors influencing health behaviors.

Responsibility II—Planning Effective Health Education Programs

Competency A: Recruit community organizations, resource people and potential participants for support and assistance in program planning.

Subcompetencies: (1) Communicate need for the program to those who will be involved. (3) Seek ideas and opinions of those who will affect, or be affected by, the program.

Competency D: Design educational programs consistent with specified program objectives.

Subcompetencies: (2) Formulate a wide variety of alternative educational methods. (3) Select strategies best suited to implementation of educational objectives in a given setting.

Responsibility III—Implementing Health Education Programs

Competency A: Exhibit competence in carrying out planned educational programs.

Subcompetencies: (1) Employ a wide range of educational methods and techniques.

Competency C: Select methods and media best suited to implement program plans for specific learners.

Subcompetencies: (1) Analyze learner characteristics, legal aspects, feasibility and other considerations influencing choices among methods.

Responsibility IV—Acting as a Resource Person in Health Education

Competency D: Select effective educational resource materials for dissemination.

Subcompetencies: (1) Assemble educational material of value to the health of individuals and community groups.

Source: National Task Force on the Preparation and Practice of Health Educators. 1985. *A competency-based curriculum for the professional preparation of entry-level health educators.* New York.

Appendix E

Overhead Masters

National Education Goals

1. Children will enter school ready to learn.

2. The high school graduation rate will be 90%.

3. Students will leave fourth, eighth and twelfth grades having showed competency in English, mathematics, science, foreign languages, civics and government, economics, arts, history and geography.

4. Teachers will have the professional development they need to help students reach the other goals.

5. American students will be first in the world in math and science achievement.

6. Every adult will be literate and have the skills to compete in the global economy and participate in American democracy.

7. Schools will be free of drugs, violence, unauthorized guns and alcohol.

8. Schools will promote partnerships with parents to increase their participation in their children's education.

Source: Hoff, D. 1994. Goals 2000 will shape state and local school reform. *Report on Education Research* 26 (12): 1–8.

Assessment and Planning Process

Step 1: Hold staff awareness meeting.

Step 2: Form assessment committee.

Step 3: Conduct assessment.

- Examine commitment to family involvement.
- Interview administrators.
- Interview teachers.
- Interview parents and other family members.
- Interview students.

Step 4: Develop assessment report.

Step 5: Present report to appropriate level of school district administration.

Step 6: Conduct action planning.

- List needs.
- Develop plan.

Step 7: Present action plan to appropriate level of school district administration.

The 8 Components of a Comprehensive School Health Program

School Health Instruction

In-class aspect of the program based on a planned and sequential curriculum. Interacts with the other components to enable young people to achieve optimal health.

Healthy School Environment

Physical and psychological surroundings of students, faculty and staff. The physical environment is free of hazards; the psychological environment fosters students' personal achievements and social growth.

School Health Services

Activities designed to appraise, protect and promote the health of students and school personnel, including preventing communicable disease and providing emergency care for injury or sudden illness.

Physical Education and Fitness

Opportunities for students to participate in daily physical activity, as well as exposure to information about how and why to partake in activities and encouragement to develop skills that contribute to lifetime fitness.

(continued...)

The 8 Components
of a Comprehensive
School Health Program
(continued)

School Nutrition and Food Services

Opportunity to establish health norms and model healthy nutritional behaviors. Schools that provide healthy food choices send a clear message to students about the importance of good nutrition.

School-Based Counseling and Personal Support

Opportunity to respond to special needs and provide personal support for students, teachers and staff, as well as promotion of schoolwide mental, emotional and social well-being.

Schoolsite Health Promotion

Combination of educational, organizational and environmental activities designed to encourage students and staff to adopt healthier lifestyles and become better consumers of health care services.

School, Family and Community Health Promotion Partnerships

Collaborative efforts that share a common vision of healthy young people and focus on health promotion and disease prevention to solve communitywide threats to the future health of youth.

Parent/Child Interaction

The interaction between parents and children may well be the most important key to lasting, long-term improvements in the overall health status of this country.

—*James O. Mason*

Educating a Child

The whole village educates the child.

—*African Proverb*

Family-Based Programs

Family-based programs theoretically have enormous potential because the family provides the most potent role models for health education, enabling change by reducing barriers and by appropriate reinforcements.

—*Cheryl Perry*

The Context for Health Education

Health education occurs in the context of family, community, religious, and media messages concerning health.

—*Maurice Elias*

Communicating with Parents

Few teacher education institutions prepare teachers to communicate with parents, even though parent involvement has been shown to have positive effects on children's achievement.

—Bermudez and Padron

Addressing Concerns About Family Involvement

Some students have no support at home and do not live in traditional family structures.

Research indicates that most parents, even those in what would be considered nontraditional family structures, want to be involved in their children's education. In some situations, other available adults (school staff, community leaders, etc.) can be used as substitutes for family members.

All parents or families will not be involved.

True, but with structured efforts the number of parents and family members involved will increase. Schools must reach out to involve as many parents as possible. Students should not be penalized in any way if their parents are not involved.

How will I find the time to plan and be involved in such programs?

Planning time is essential for parent and family involvement activities. With limited planning time, efforts to increase parent involvement may have to start out on a small scale and gradually increase over time. The school district commitment to family involvement must include providing time for teacher preparation and planning.

What about the district administration? Will they support us?

Administrative support is absolutely necessary. School districts should develop a family involvement policy and/or strategic plan that specifically identifies the role of the school administration relative to program support.

Many of my student's parents speak a different language. How can I communicate with them?

For in-person meetings with parents, if necessary, a translator should be available. Written materials should be written in English and other appropriate languages. Schools can also form advisory committees to address ways of improving communication.

References

Airhihenbuwa, C. O. 1990. A conceptual model for cultural appropriate health education programs in developing countries. *International Quarterly of Community Health Education* 11:53-72.

Allensworth, D. D. 1994. Health education: State of the art. *Journal of School Health* 63 (1): 14-20.

Bartell, J. F. 1992. Starting from scratch. *Principal* 72:13-14.

Bensley, L. B. 1994. Staff development for multicultural competency. In *The multicultural challenge in health education,* ed. A. C. Matiella, 267-295. Santa Cruz, CA: ETR Associates.

Bermudez, A. B., and Y. N. Padron. 1986. University-school collaboration that increases minority parent involvement. *Educational Horizons* 66 (2): 83-86.

Bernier, M. P. 1991. Parental involvement in health education. *The Eta Sigma Gamma Monograph Series* 9 (1): 42-48.

Birch, D. A. 1992. Improving leadership skills in curriculum development. *Journal of School Health* 62 (1): 27-28.

Boschee, F. 1988. Comprehensive school health: Directives for development and implementation. *Health Education* 19 (5): 36-38.

Chavkin, N. F. 1989. A multicultural perspective on parent involvement: Implications for policy and practice. *Education* 109 (3): 276-285.

Chavkin, N. F., and D. L. Williams. 1985. *Executive summary of the final report: Parent involvement in education project.* Austin, TX: Southwest Educational Development Laboratory.

Chavkin, N. F., and D. L. Williams. 1988. Critical issues in teacher training for parent involvement. *Educational Horizons* 66:87-89.

Chavkin, N. F., and D. L. Williams. 1990. Working parents: Implications for practice. *Education* 111 (2): 242-248.

Comer, J. P. 1991. Parent participation: Fad or function. *Educational Horizons* 69 (4): 182-188.

Cooper, K., and M. L. Gonzalez. 1993. Communicating with parents when you don't speak their language. *Principal* 73 (2): 45-46.

Criteria for comprehensive health education curricula. 1989. Los Alamitos, CA: Southwest Regional Education Laboratory.

Davies, D. 1991. Schools reaching out. *Phi Delta Kappan* 72 (5): 376-382.

Delgado-Gaitan, C. 1991. Involving parents in the schools: A process of empowerment. *American Journal of Education* 100:20-26.

Elias, M. J. 1990. The role of affect and social relationships in health behavior and school health curriculum and instruction. *Journal of School Health* 60 (4): 157-163.

Epps, V. 1987. Teacher initiatives that lead to quality health education programs. *Health Education* 18 (5): 44-47.

Epstein, J. 1993. Make parents your partners. *Instructor* 102 (8): 52-53.

Fetro, J. 1992. *Personal and social skills: Understanding and integrating competencies across health content.* Santa Cruz, CA: ETR Associates.

Figueroa, J. 1993. Can parental involvement and bilingual education save our language minority children from becoming disempowered and disenfranchised? *Illinois School Journal* 72 (2): 40-49.

The FIRST grants. 1992. *Phi Delta Kappan* 72 (5): 383-388.

Flaxman, E., and M. Inger. 1992. Parents and schooling in the 1990s. *Education Digest* 57:3-7.

Hawkins, J. D., and R. F. Catalano. 1990. Broadening the vision of education: Schools as health promoting environments. *Journal of School Health* 60 (4): 178-181.

Heleen, O. 1992. Is your school family friendly? *Principal* 72 (2): 5-7.

Henderson, A. T. 1987. *The evidence continues to grow: Parent involvement improves student achievement.* Columbia, MD: National Committee for Citizens in Education.

Herman, B. E. 1993. Parents' choice. *The American School Board Journal* 180 (2): 46.

Hern, M., et al. 1992. Involving families in cardiovascular health promotion: The CATCH feasibility study. *Journal of Health Education* 23 (1): 22-31.

Hernandez, M. E., and C. A. Day. 1994. Family involvement in the classroom and school site. In *The multicultural challenge in health education,* ed. A. C. Matiella, 331-357. Santa Cruz, CA: ETR Associates.

Hoff, D. 1994. Goals 2000 will shape state and local school reform. *Report on Education Research* 26 (12): 1-8.

Howard-Hamilton, M. 1992. Facilitative communication: The end of the beginning. In *Valuing diversity: Bridging the gap through interpersonal skills,* ed. J. Wittmer, 247-255. Minneapolis, MN: Educational Media Corporation.

Iammarino, N. K., A. D. Weinberg, L. Laufman and H. P. Cooper. 1992. Family history as educational construct in cardiovascular education. *Wellness Perspectives: Research, Theory and Practice* 8 (3): 3-18.

Kane, W. 1993. *Step by step to comprehensive school health: The program planning guide.* Santa Cruz, CA: ETR Associates.

Kirschenbaum, H. 1982. Handling school-community controversies over health education curriculum. *Health Education* 13:7-10.

Mason, J. O. 1989. Forging working partnerships for school health education. *Journal of School Health* 59 (1): 18-20.

McKenzie, J., and M. K. Beyrer. 1979. Checkpoints for developing an in-house curriculum. *Health Education* 10:14-16.

Morrow, R. 1991. The challenge of Southeast Asian parental involvement. *Principal* 70 (4): 20-21.

Nadar, P. R., et al. 1989. A family approach to cardiovascular risk reduction: Results from the San Diego family health project. *Health Education Quarterly* 16 (2): 229-244.

National Task Force on the Preparation and Practice of Health Educators. 1985. *A competency-based curriculum for the professional preparation of entry-level health educators.* New York.

Pahnos, M. L., and K. L. Butt. Integrating multicultural health education into the curriculum. In *The multicultural challenge in health education,* ed. A. C. Matiella, 133-149. Santa Cruz, CA: ETR Associates.

The parent factor. 1991. *American School Board Journal* 178:A1-27.

Perry, C. L., S. J. Crockett and P. Pirie. 1987. Influencing parental health behavior: Implications of community assessments. *Health Education* 18 (5): 68-77.

Perry, C. L., R. V. Luepker, D. M. Murray, C. Kurth, R. Mullia, S. Crockett and D. R. Jacobs. 1988. Parent involvement with children's health promotion: The Minnesota home team. *American Journal of Public Health* 78 (9): 1156-1160.

Pollack, M. 1987. *Planning and implementing health education in schools.* Mountain View, CA: Mayfield Publishing Associates.

Radd, T. 1993. Restructuring parent-teacher organizations to increase parental influence on the educational process. *Elementary School Guidance and Counseling* 27 (4): 280-287.

Roberts, L. C. 1982. Regardless of race: Toward communication free of racial and ethnic bias. In *Without bias: A guidebook for non-discriminatory communication,* 2d ed., ed. J. C. Pickens, 4-22. New York: Wiley.

Usdansky, M. 1994. More kids live in changing family. *USA Today,* 30 April.

Walberg, H. 1984. Families as partners in educational productivity. *Phi Delta Kappan* 65:397-400.

Werch, C., M. Young, M. Clark, C. Garrett, S. Hooks and C. Kersten. 1991. Effects of a take home drug prevention program on drug-related communication and beliefs of parents and children. *Journal of School Health* 61 (8): 346-350.

Wisconsin Department of Public Instruction. 1985. *A guide to curriculum planning in health education.* Madison, WI.